Language: English

These materials are designed to assist you in learning about hope. They should not be used for medical advice, counseling, or other health-related services. iFred, The Shine Hope Company and Kathryn Goetzke do not endorse or provide any medical advice, diagnosis, or treatment. The information provided herein should not be used for the diagnosis or treatment of any medical condition and cannot be substituted for the advice of physicians, licensed professionals, or therapists who are familiar with your specific situation. Consult a licensed medical professional, or call 911, if you are in need of immediate assistance.

ISBN: 979-8-9884988-1-0

WELCOME TO
Hopeful Mindsets®
on the College Campus

Thank you for participating in the Hopeful Mindsets on the College Campus course. This is the first step on your hope journey. Hope is a teachable, measurable, and learnable skill that can have positive ramifications on every aspect of your life.

This course cannot make you hopeful; however, it can teach you the "how-to" of hope by helping you incorporate critical hope skills into your daily routine. Each lesson of this course will provide you with video and text lessons, workbook reflections, and weekly actions that are all designed to help you create, maintain, and grow hope.

As you go through each lesson, you can use the corresponding pages of this coursebook to reflect on your hope journey and continue to reinforce the skills you learn. Remember, your hope journey is up to you. The more you use the coursebook pages, lessons, videos, and resources provided, the stronger your hopeful mindset will become.

Welcome to the Hopeful Mindsets community.

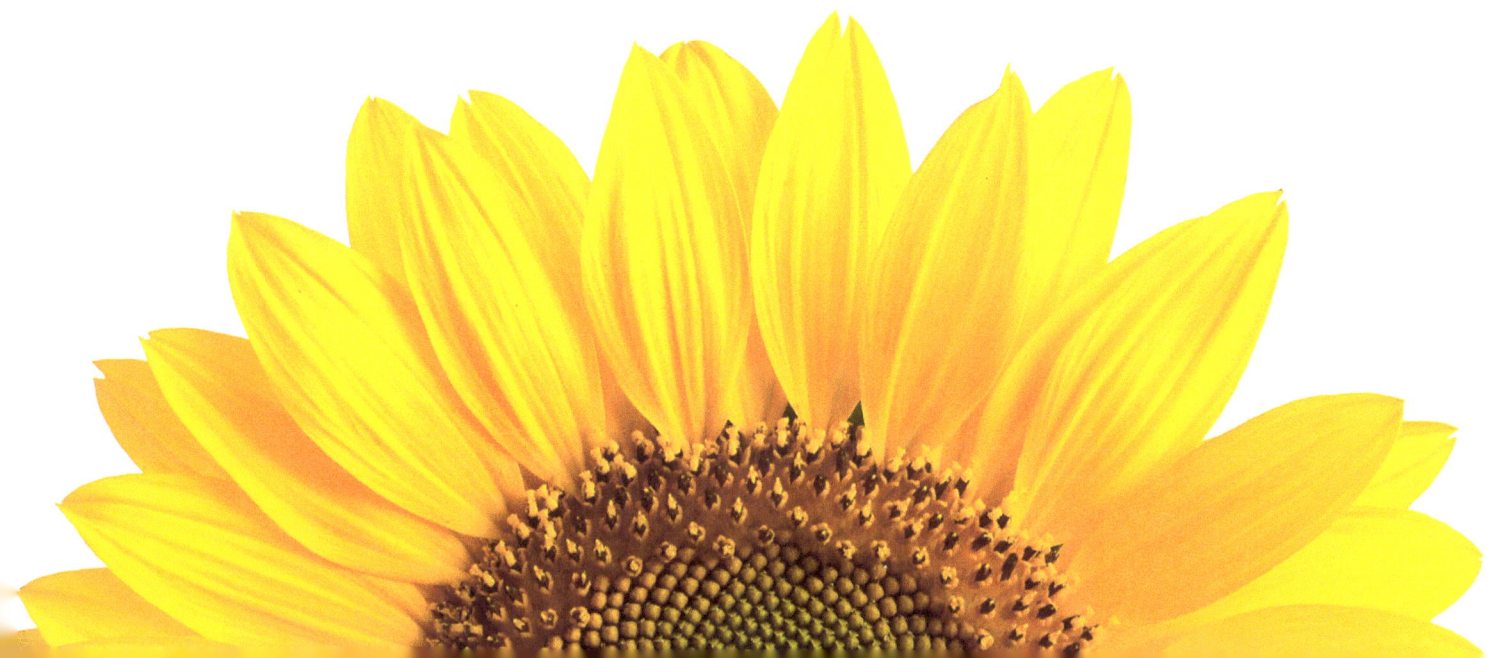

We would like to thank the following people for their contribution to our programs:

This program would not be possible without the brilliant leadership, support, and commitment to hope by:

Myron L. Belfer MD, MPA, Harvard Catalyst
Myron is Professor of Psychiatry in the Department of Psychiatry, Children's Hospital Boston, Harvard Medical School, and Senior Associate in Psychiatry at the Children's Hospital of Boston. Dr. Belfer is a Champion for Hope.

Kathryn Goetzke MBA, Author, Creator
Contributors: Taylor Steed, Katharine Lee-Kramer, Veronica O'Brien
Sarah Mellen, Mic Fariscal, Anna Termulo Montances and **Naneth Samoya-Jumawid**

To our advisors, hope contributors, and experts:
Dr. Edward Barksdale, Dr. Frank Gard Jameson, Mayor Hillary Schieve, Kristy L. Stark M.A., Ed.M., BCBA, Karen Kirby PhD, MSc, BSc, C.Psychol, AfBPS, SFHEA, Ulster University, **Marie Dunne and the Northern Ireland** team that helped plant the seeds for this work.

Pioneers in early Hope Science including **Dr. Crystal Bryce, Dr. Dan Tomasulo, Dr. Chan Hellman, Dr. Matthew Gallagher, Dr. Jennifer Cheavens** and the late **Dr. Shane Lopez.**

iFred Board of Directors:
Tom Dean, Susan Minamyer, Jim Link, Dr. John Grohol, Kathryn Goetzke, Dr. Mindy Magrane

The Hopeful Minds Advisory Board

Some of our early funders: Sutter Health, Anthem, The Gordon Family Giving Fund of the Parasol Tahoe Community Foundation, The Shine Hope Company, and The Mood Factory.

IN SPECIAL RECOGNITION
Susan Minamyer, whose unconditional love, support, encouragement, faith, and brilliance planted and watered the seeds necessary to create and grow this program. Kathryn's big brothers **Arnold and Fred, and Clara, Maura, Jack, Sophie, Charles, and Sarah,** who continue to strengthen, build, and inspire Kathryn's hope.

IN HONOR
In recognition of all in the world that struggled with hopelessness in some way, shape or form, and left us way too early, including a few close to our hearts. Thank you for teaching us so much about life, love, and hope. May we spread Hope far and wide in your name and honor:
Jon and Sally Goetzke, Tom Foorman, Dr. Stephen C. Gleason, Vicky Harrison, Eloise Land, Jesse Lewis, and Austin Weirich.

TABLE OF CONTENTS

DEFINITION LIST

The most important terms we use in our Coursebook, and that we hope you will start using, include:

HOPE: We define hope as a vision for something in the future, fueled by both positive feelings and inspired actions.

HOPELESSNESS: Hopelessness is both a feeling of despair and a sense of helplessness. It is emotional (a negative feeling) and motivational (an inability to act). We all experience moments of hopelessness and manage them with hope skills.

POSITIVE FEELINGS: Positive feelings are those feelings that help us to stay hopeful as we work towards our goals.

INSPIRED ACTIONS: Inspired actions are the deliberate steps you take to get in your upstairs brains and toward your goals in life.

UPSTAIRS BRAIN: This is where our thinking, imagining, problem-solving, and learning occur. This part of the brain is responsible for the development of sound decision-making and planning, control over emotions and body, and self-understanding and empathy. The upstairs brain is also where we access our positive feelings.

DOWNSTAIRS BRAIN: Also referred to as the reptilian brain, this part of the brain is responsible for basic functions such as breathing, blinking, heart rate, and fight, flight, freeze, or fawn mode. It is also responsible for the chemical stimulus associated with strong emotions, such as anger, sadness, and fear.

STRESS RESPONSE: Your stress response is when an external or internal trigger causes your brain to release stress hormones, such as cortisol, adrenaline, and norepinephrine, that force you into your fight, flight, freeze, or fawn mode. It generally lasts 90 seconds from time of the last trigger.

STRESS SKILLS: These are actions that help you navigate your stress response and work through your body's chemical response to external stimuli, to get manage your downstairs brain and get you back upstairs.

HAPPINESS HABITS: These are healthy, long-term habits that help you stay in your upstairs brain, where you access the problem-solving skills, collaboration, and passion, all critical for hope. When you take time for Happiness Habits, your brain releases happiness hormones, such as endorphins, dopamine, serotonin, and oxytocin.

NOURISHING NETWORKS: Your Nourishing Networks are the Hope Networks of the people in your life that provide you with support, help you stay on track, encourage you to succeed, and who you do the same for in return.

ELIMINATING CHALLENGES: Challenges to Hope are negative thinking patterns, like limiting beliefs, automatic negative thoughts, all-or-nothing thinking, negative bias, rumination, worry, focusing on uncontrollables, attaching to outcomes, and internalizing failure, that can keep us in hopelessness states. Eliminating challenges are the conscious act of using hope skills to overcome these challenges and get back to hope.

THE HOPE MATRIX™: The Hope Matrix is the process that we use to get from hopelessness to hope. The Hope Matrix teaches us that to cultivate hope, we must move from despair to positive feelings, and from helplessness to inspired actions.

Shine Hope™: This is the mnemonic we use to remember our hope skills. Shine stands for: **S**tress Skills, **H**appiness Habits, **I**nspired Actions, **N**ourishing Networks, and **E**liminating Challenges and is what we use to activate skills for hope.

THE HOPE MATRIX

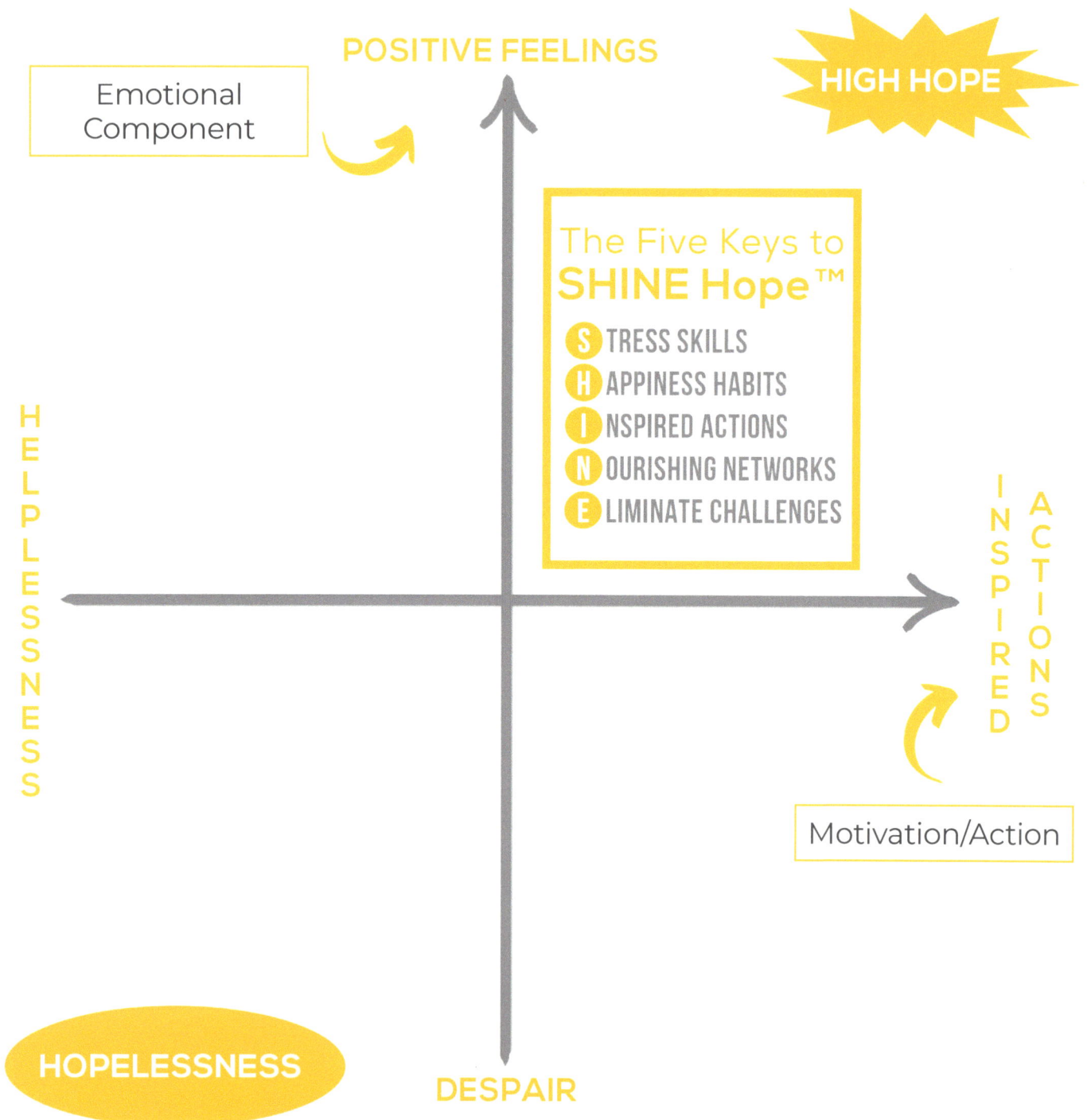

POSITIVE FEELINGS

Emotional Component

HIGH HOPE

The Five Keys to SHINE Hope™

- **S**TRESS SKILLS
- **H**APPINESS HABITS
- **I**NSPIRED ACTIONS
- **N**OURISHING NETWORKS
- **E**LIMINATE CHALLENGES

HELPLESSNESS

INSPIRED ACTIONS

Motivation/Action

HOPELESSNESS

DESPAIR

PREPARATION DAY

As you prepare for your Hopeful Mindsets course, take time to reflect on how hope will improve your life. What are the outcomes you want to see? How do you want to feel and interact with hope on a daily basis? How will a hopeful mindset help you face challenges throughout your college career?

Before Lesson 1 of the course begins, watch the Preparation Day Video and complete the following prompts:

MEASURE HOPE

Your hope score is a tool for you to use to monitor your progress, track your hope journey, and reflect on how hopeful you are in the current moment. Hope is not fixed; when you practice hope skills, you can improve your hope score.

Use the link provided to take the Snyder Hope Scale Assessment or scan QR code:
theshinehopecompany.com/measure-your-hope/

My Current Snyder Hope Scale Score: _____

Why do you measure hope?

_____

_____

How do you feel about your score?

_____

_____

How hopeful have you been in life?

_____

_____

In what areas of your life do you feel like you could be more hopeful?

_____

_____

How has your hope impacted your ability to achieve goals?

_____

_____

This course teaches you the hope skills you can use to create, maintain, and grow hope. No matter what hope score you received, the goal of this course is to learn the "how-to" of hope both for yourself and others. This course is not only a model for your own life; it is a framework you can use to share the power of hope with others.

Who in your life could benefit from higher hope?

_____

_____

What organizations or businesses in your community could benefit from learning about hope?

_____

_____

IDENTIFYING YOUR STRENGTHS

Understanding your strengths is important for creating and maintaining hope. Focusing on your strengths can help you manage your stress response, cultivate positive thoughts, and focus on the future. As you continue though this workbook, you will repeatedly be asked to reflect on your strengths.

Take a moment to learn more about your strengths by taking the free VIA Character Strengths Survey here or scan QR Code:

theshinehopecompany.pro.viasurvey.org

Write down the top five strengths identified in your results:

1 _____

2 _____

3 _____

4 _____

5 _____

Which of these strengths do you think is most tied to your ability to maintain hope?

_____

_____

Are you activating your strengths regularly? How so?

_____

_____

How can you better utilize your strengths at home? In school?

_____

_____

PREPARING FOR THE COURSE

You are 95% more likely to achieve your goal if you write it down and regularly touch base with a friend.

As you will learn in this course, goals are an important component of a Hopeful Mindset. By measuring your hope levels, creating a SMART Goal for hope, and finding a friend that you can check in with after each lesson, you will be increasing the benefits that you will gain from this course.

What are you most looking forward to about this course?

_____

_____

Identify one SMART Goal you have for the course *(SMART Goals are goals that are* **S***pecific,* **M***easurable,* **A***chievable,* **R***elevant, and* **T***imebound):*

_____

_____

List three obstacles that could stop you from finishing this course

1 _____

2 _____

3 _____

How can you overcome these obstacles?

_____

_____

Identify a friend to check in with after each lesson:

_____

I asked my friend, and they are willing to play this roll: YES

Identify Your Limiting Beliefs

Information about the following section can be found under "The Power of Belief" in Lesson 1 of this course.

Limiting beliefs are subconscious thoughts that appear through negative emotions, anxiety, and self-doubt. You can identify your limiting beliefs by asking yourself these questions:

What are the results you've produced in your life that you're proud of?

_____

Where are your results not in alignment with what you really want to be, do, or have?

_____

What area of your life have you really tried to improve but, no matter what, things just didn't get better?

_____

In these areas where the results you are seeing aren't what you are hoping for, there is a good chance that you are being plagued by limiting beliefs.

Write down three limiting beliefs you have about yourself, hope, and college.

1 Identify three limiting beliefs you have about yourself:

Examples: _I am not smart enough; I can't do anything right; I am not worthy; I always fail; I have no power to improve my life; I am incapable of change_

1. _____

2. _____

3. _____

2 Identify three limiting beliefs you have about hope:

Examples: *Hope leads to disappointment; Hope leads to failure; I cannot affect the amount of hope I have in my life; I will always be hopeless*

1. _____

2. _____

3. _____

3 Identify three limiting beliefs you have about college:

Examples: *I can't graduate; I'm not smart enough to be here; I am going to fail*

1. _____

2. _____

3. _____

Questioning Limiting Beliefs

Byron Katie's process of self-inquiry, called "The Work" invites you to ask four questions about each limiting belief you encounter:

1. Is it true?
2. Can you absolutely know that it's true?
3. How do you react when you believe that thought?
4. Who would you be without the thought?

As you answer each of these questions, you can begin to see how the thought is limiting your true potential.

For three of the limiting beliefs you identified, answer Byron Katie's four questions:

Limiting Belief #1: _____

Is it true? _____

Can you absolutely know that it's true? _____

How do you react when you believe that thought?

_____

Who would you be without that thought?

_____

Limiting Belief #2: _____

Is it true? _____

Can you absolutely know that it's true? _____

How do you react when you believe that thought?

_____

Who would you be without that thought?

_____

Limiting Belief #3: _____

Is it true? _____

Can you absolutely know that it's true? _____

How do you react when you believe that thought?

_____

Who would you be without that thought?

_____

Challenge Your Beliefs with Thoughts and Actions

Your limiting beliefs are only beliefs; they are not truths. Try overcoming a limiting belief by focusing on an opposite, reaffirming belief. Take action to make this new belief a reality.

Write out the nine limiting beliefs you identified, and then a reaffirming belief to replace each one with:

Examples of reaffirming beliefs for myself:
I am smart enough; I am worthy; I am I have the power to improve my life

Examples of reaffirming beliefs for hope:
I am worthy of hope; hope is teachable; hope can improve all areas of my life

Examples of reaffirming beliefs for college:
I deserve to be in college; I can manage my college experience; I am smart enough to graduate from college

Limiting Beliefs:

_____

_____

_____

_____

_____

_____

Reaffirming Beliefs:

_____

_____

_____

_____

_____

_____

The Hope Matrix™

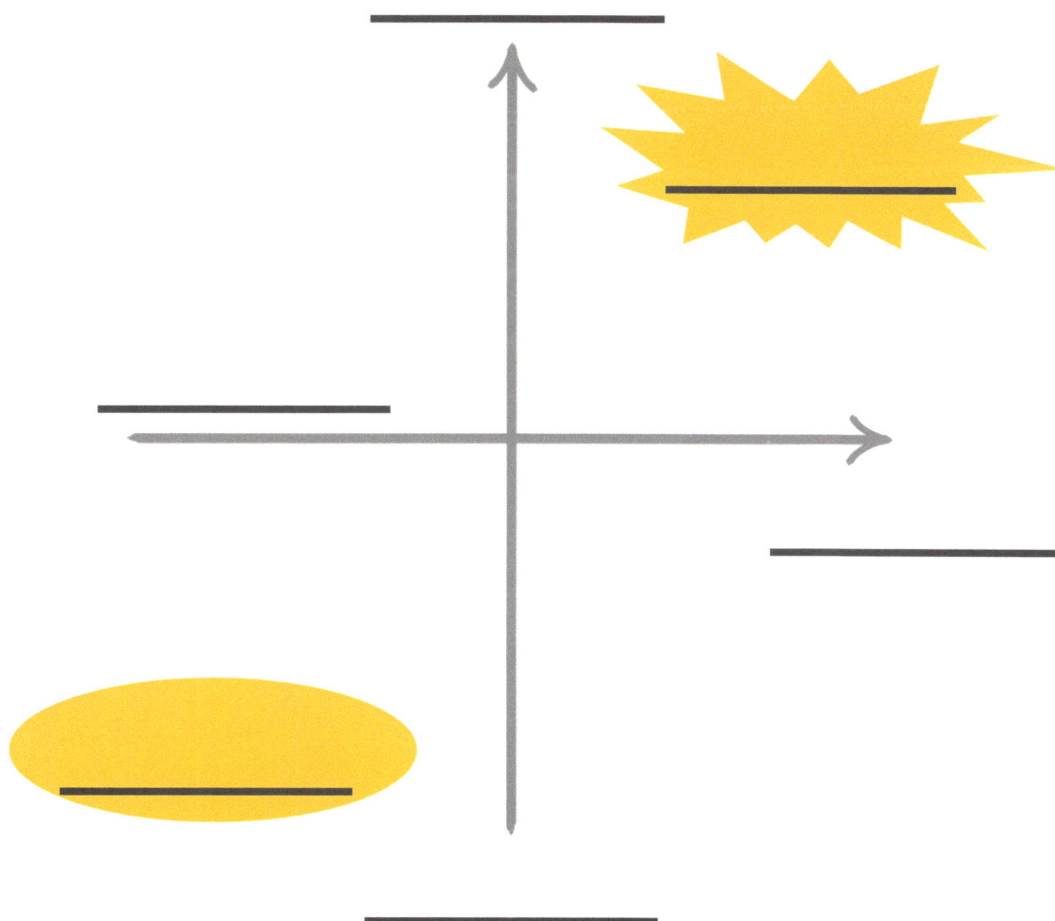

The Hope Matrix is a tool that illustrates how to manage hopelessness and get to hope. By proactively managing our despair and helplessness, no matter what life brings, we can find our way from hopelessness to hope.

Directions: Fill in the blanks below with the following words: Hope, Hopelessness, Despair, Helplessness, Positive Feelings, Inspired Actions.

Lesson 1 Inspired Action

Reaffirm your positive beliefs about yourself, your hope, and your college experience to prepare for the rest of the course. Identify the three most important reaffirming beliefs above. Take time to tell yourself these reaffirming beliefs at least three times each day. Be sure to notice what you say to yourself normally, and how saying something new feels.

Lesson 1 Friend Check in:

Did you check in with your Hopeful   YES   NO
Mindsets friend today?

What did you discuss with them? Did they provide any interesting insights about this lesson?

_____

_____

Did they identify limiting beliefs surrounding themselves, their hope, or their college experience? How were they similar to yours? How were they different?

_____

_____

Did they have any reaffirming beliefs? What reaffirming beliefs will help you most in this course?

_____

_____

How will checking in with your friend help you meet your goals?

_____

_____

Lesson 2: **THE SCIENCE OF HOPE**
COURSE REFLECTION

Your daily coursebook reflection today gives you time to reflect on what hope means to you, and what you are hopeful for in your personal life, school/work life, and for your health and wellness.

Read the Lesson 2 text and watch the Lesson 2 Hopeful Mindsets course videos, then answer the questions below:

What is your definition of hope?

_____

_____

Does your definition of hope include both feelings (emotional) and actions (motivational)?

_____

_____

Why is action an important component of hope?

_____

_____

How can hope impact your life?

_____

_____

What are you hopeful for in the following areas of your life:

Personal Life:

_____

College:

_____

Work:

_____

Relationships:

_____

Health and Wellness:

_____

Community:

_____

What areas of your life are in most need of hope?

_____

_____

Think of a time in your life when you had low hope in a specific area. What strategies did you use to increase hope?

_____

_____

Identify people in your life that add to your hope.

_____

_____

Lesson 2 Inspired Action

Reflect on the coursebook questions throughout the week. Are there other areas of your life where you have high or low hope? Did you identify other things in your life that you are hopeful for? Note your findings in the reflections.

Remember- the more you can identify areas of hopefulness and hopelessness in your life, the easier it will be to use hope skills to activate hope in your life. Taking time each day to reflect on these questions builds an important foundation for your hope journey.

Lesson 2 Friend Check in:

Did you check in with your Hopeful   YES   NO
Mindsets friend today?

What did you discuss with them? Did they provide any interesting insights about this lesson?

_____

_____

What strategies are you both going to do to increase hope in the areas of your lives you feel are lacking hope?

_____

_____

Share what strategies have helped you both in the past.

_____

_____

Lesson 3: **THE IMPACT OF HOPELESSNESS**
COURSE REFLECTION

Read the Lesson 3 text and watch the Lesson 3 Hopeful Mindsets course videos, then answer the questions below:

Hopelessness Reflection

Everyone feels hopeless at times throughout their lives. It is therefore important that you develop the skills you need to address hopelessness and return to a hopeful mindset.

Take time to reflect on the following prompts and answer them as fully and honestly as possible:

What is your definition of hopelessness?

_____

_____

Does it include both emotions (feelings, such as despair) and motivations (such as helplessness)?

_____

_____

Our experts recognize that when they are hopeless they feel sad and overwhelmed, and experience physical responses, such as a lack of appetite or trouble getting out of bed. What does hopelessness look like in your life?

_____

_____

_____

_____

Identifying Your Feelings

Using the questions below, think about the last time you experienced each of the three emotions associated with despair, and start to explore how you feel these emotions and express them.

ANGER

Describe the last time you were angry:

_____

How did you experience anger in your mind?   _____

How did you experience anger in your body?   _____

How did you respond when you were angry?

_____

What did your anger tell you about your environment or yourself?

_____

What are unhealthy ways you respond to anger?   _____

What are healthy ways you respond to anger?   _____

SADNESS

Describe the last time you were sad:

_____

How did you experience sadness in your mind?   _____

How did you experience sadness in your body?   _____

How did you respond when you were sad?

_____

What did your sadness tell you about your environment or yourself?

_____

What are unhealthy ways you respond to sadness?
                                                _____

What are healthy ways you respond to sadness?   _____

FEAR

Describe the last time you were afraid:

_____

How did you experience fear in your mind?   _____

How did you experience fear in your body?   _____

How did you respond when you were afraid?

_____

What did your fear tell you about your environment or yourself?

_____

What are unhealthy ways you respond to fear?
                                             _____

What are healthy ways you respond to fear?   _____

Managing Hopelessness

Describe a specific situation in the past when you felt hopeless. What emotional strategies did you use to get back to hope? What motivational (action) strategies did you use to get out of helplessness?

_____

_____

_____

_____

What did the situation teach you?

_____

_____

_____

_____

Can you identify anyone that helped or hurt you in managing this hopelessness?

_____

_____

Describe something you feel hopeless about right now. What emotional strategies are you using to get back to hope? What motivational (action) strategies are you using to get out of helplessness?

_____

_____

_____

_____

Who is someone you can turn to for help?

_____

_____

Think of a time when you may feel hopeless in college in the future. What is an emotional strategy you will be able to use to get back to hope? What is a motivational (action) strategy you will be able to use to get out of helplessness?

_____

_____

_____

_____

Who is someone you will be able to turn to for help?

_____

_____

_____

_____

Resources for Hope on Campus

When our stress response is activated or we are experiencing hopelessness, we can't access our problem-solving capabilities in our upstairs brain. It is therefore important to know about the resources available to you before you or someone you know needs them.

Identifying the resources available isn't just about preparing yourself. It is also about being able to help others. By filling out the Resources for Hope on Campus poster on the next page and posting it somewhere on campus, you can help your fellow students find the resources they need when they are struggling.

This is how we are proactive about hope. Did we forget to list anything? Send us an e-mail at support@theshinehopecompany.com

RESOURCES FOR HOPE ON CAMPUS

CAMPUS COUNSELING CENTER

Location: _____

Hours: _____

Phone Number: _____

LOCAL CRISIS HOTLINE

Phone Number: _____

Text Number: _____

Hours: _____

HEALTH CENTER

Location: _____

Hours: _____

Phone Number: _____

CAMPUS POLICE

Location: _____

Hours: _____

Phone Number: _____

COUNSELING CENTER

Location: _____

Hours: _____

Phone Number: _____

DISABILITY RESOURCE CENTER

Location: _____

Hours: _____

Phone Number: _____

FINANCIAL AID OFFICE

Location: _____

Hours: _____

Phone Number: _____

FOOD RESOURCES ORGANIZATION

Location: _____

Hours: _____

Phone Number: _____

TUTORING SUPPORT

Location: _____

Hours: _____

Phone Number: _____

ADDICTION SUPPORT

Location: _____

Hours: _____

Phone Number: _____

CAMPUS GYM

Location: _____

Hours: _____

Phone Number: _____

OTHER RECREATION AREAS:

_____

_____

_____

OTHER RESOURCES AVAILABLE

_____

_____

_____

Hopeful Mindsets®
on the College Campus

SCAN FOR OTHER RESOURCES

Lesson 3 Inspired Action

Begin to identify the times when you experience hopelessness. Where does hopelessness show up for you, in your mind, and body? Remember: if you want to proactively manage your hopelessness, then awareness of when, where, and how you experience it is the first step.

Lesson 3 Friend Check in:

Did you check in with your Hopeful   YES   NO
Mindsets friend today?

What did you discuss with them? Did they provide any interesting insights about this lesson?

_____

_____

What was one time that they felt hopeless? How did they overcome it?

_____

_____

Were they able to identify other ways you could overcome the past, current, or future feelings of hopelessness you identified?

_____

_____

SHINE HOPE™

A HOW-TO FOR HOPE IN TRYING TIMES

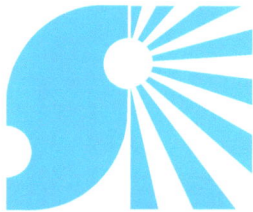

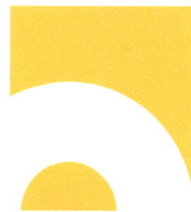

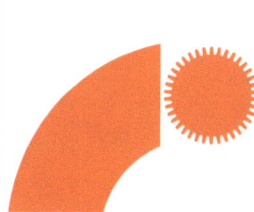

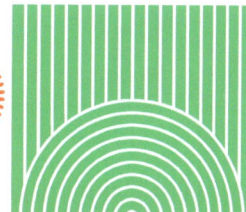

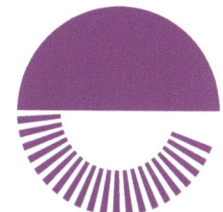

S TRESS SKILLS	**H** APPINESS HABITS	**I** NSPIRED ACTIONS	**N** OURISHING NETWORKS	**E** LIMINATING CHALLENGES
90 second pause	Activating purpose	WOOP process	5:1 Rule	Limiting beliefs
Belly breathing	Pursuing passion	SMART goals	Compassion	Automatic Negative Thoughts (ANTs)
Journaling	Utilizing strengths	Stretch goals	Forgiveness	All-or-nothing thinking
Gardening	Meditation	Achievement goals	Love	Negative bias
Calming music	Smiling	Intrinsic goals	Gratitude	Rumination & Worry
Affirming beliefs	Exercising / Nutrition	Mastery goals	Recognition	Focusing on Uncontrollables
Sensory engagement	Creating / listening to music	Micro goals / Stepping	Support	Attaching to outcomes
Cold plunge	Dancing / Singing	Habit Stacking	Faith	Internalizing failure
Decluttering	Drawing / Painting	Visualization	Trust	Toxic Consumption
Prayer	Gratitude	Overcoming obstacles	Respect	Nocebo Effect
Nature walk	Volunteering	Regoaling	Effective Listening	Mind Wandering
Napping	Wonder / Awe	Write down goals / check in	Empathy	Implicity Bias
Laughter	Quality sleep		Kindness	Negative Framing
Crying	Doodling		Animals	Perfectionism
Tapping				Taking things personally
Yoga				
Mantras				

the shine hope™ company

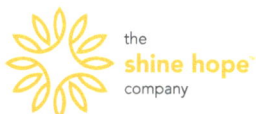

Scan the QR Code to measure hope with the Hope Scale!

STRESS SKILLS

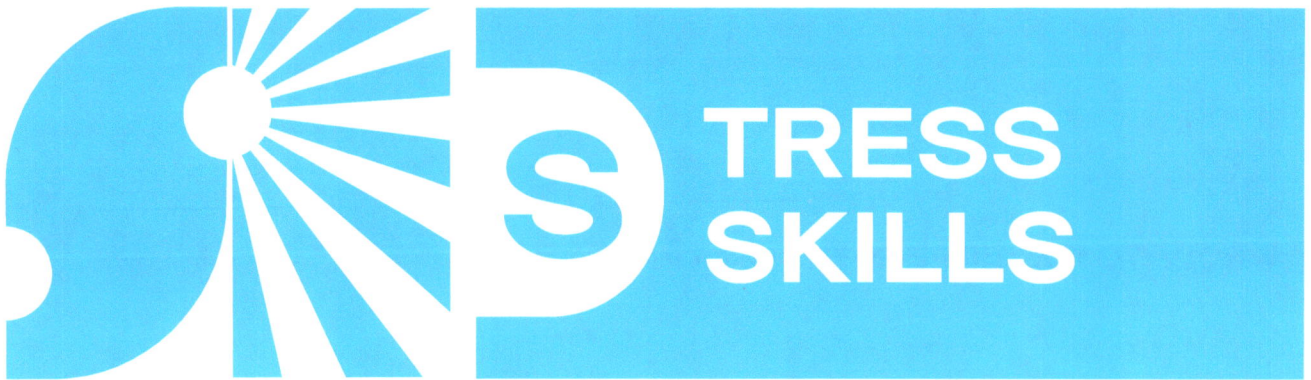

Stress Skills are actions that help you navigate your stress response and work through your body's chemical response to external stimuli. By practicing them, you are teaching yourself how to proactively manage the emotional despair found in hopelessness and move towards positive feelings where you activate hope.

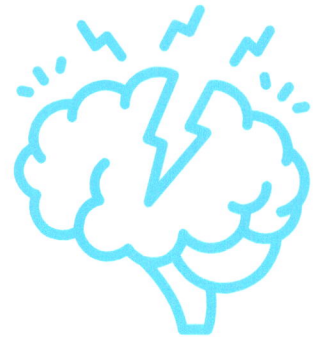

The Stress Response

This is when you are emotionally triggered by something in your environment, and you go into fight, flight, freeze, or fawn mode as your body releases stress hormones, such as cortisol, adrenaline, and norepinephrine. You are in your downstairs brain, and can't reach your upstairs brain; the upstairs brain is the place where you make good decisions for moving towards all you hope for in life.

90 second pause	Sensory engagement	Laughter
Belly breathing	Cold plunge	Crying
Journaling	Decluttering	Tapping
Gardening	Prayer	Yoga
Calming music	Nature walk	Mantras
Affirming beliefs	Napping	

Lesson 4: **STRESS SKILLS**
COURSE REFLECTION

Read the Lesson 4 text and watch the Lesson 4 Hopeful Mindsets course videos, then answer the questions below:

The First Key to Shine Hope

The First Key to Shine Hope is Identifying and Managing Your Stress Response.

What is your stress response and how do you identify it?
_____
_____

How long does it take the stress response to cycle through your body?
_____
_____

Think of a time in the past week when you were stressed. How did you feel the stress in your brain? Your body?
_____
_____

Did you work to decrease your stress response? What did you do? Did it work? Why or why not?
_____
_____

When you noticed your stress response, what did you think? Did you have limiting beliefs? How did your thoughts, positive or negative, impact your stress response?

_____
_____

Chronic stress is a prolonged state of stress, anxiety, or fear that can be debilitating and often impacts multiple areas in our life. Have you experienced chronic stress in the past? Are you currently experiencing it? Take some time to reflect on times when you have experienced chronic stress and think about what prolonged your stress. How might you release that stress? What actions can you take to relieve that stress?

_____

_____

_____

_____

Trigger Worksheet

One of the greatest barriers to hope is found in the First Key to Shine Hope: Identifying and Managing the Stress Response. When stress is at an all-time high, we are much more reactive than normal. It is important to learn what is triggering us, and start unwinding this process so we can respond in healthy ways. In Lesson 3, we worked on identifying sadness, fear, and anger and how we react to these emotions. When you identify one of these emotions during your day, the next step is to reflect on what triggered the emotion.

Over the next week, take time each day to add to the Trigger Worksheet on the next page. Triggers are sometimes hard to spot unless they are really big. Yet by keeping a regular account, you start to see what areas you need to work on, and what specifically you can do about it. You can also start to see how your stress response affects your body and brain and how you can begin to proactively manage your response using Stress Skills and respond in healthy ways that bring you back to a positive mindset.

Trigger Worksheet

TRIGGER	LIMITING BELIEF	EMOTION FELT	WHERE IN MY BODY IS IT FELT	MY BEHAVIOR/ RESPONSE	STRESS SKILL I CAN USE	RESOLUTION TO TRIGGER EVENT
EXAMPLES						
Did poorly on quiz	I am a failure	Fear, shame	Stomach	Shut down, lose motivation to try	Deep breathing	I created a plan to stay on top of my coursework

Influencing Our Emotional Response

This exercise is an excerpt from Dr. Dan Tomasulo's book, *"Learned Hopefulness."* It can help you to understand how the negative emotions you encounter during your stress response can be shifted towards positive feelings. Research shows that feelings of hope and optimism result from reframing past experiences.

Write about one moment in your life when a negative event led to unforeseen positive circumstances. Important things were lost, but other opportunities presented themselves that otherwise may not have. You could have closed the door, or it could have been closed on you. The important thing is that the second door could not have opened unless the first one closed.

_____

_____

_____

_____

Reflect on your example. Write about the circumstances that surrounded the event. If something like that happened now, would you respond differently? What positive things emerged? Were there actions you took that helped bring about the positive development?

_____

_____

_____

_____

This can be a great way to manage your emotions and learn hopefulness. We see how dark situations in our lives have transformed into something positive. Instead of seeing only challenges when we are triggered, we now know firsthand that other difficulties turned out better than expected.

Identifying Stress Skills

Stress Skills are actions that help you navigate your stress response and work through your body's chemical response to external stimuli. By practicing them, you are teaching yourself how to proactively manage the emotional despair found in hopelessness and move towards positive feelings where you activate hope.

Some examples of short-term Stress Skills include:

- Taking a 90-Second Pause (The Clear Button)
- Deep breathing
- Being aware of feelings
- Listening to calming music
- Engaging your five senses to get present
- Any other skill that helps you navigate your 90-second stress response

Some Examples of long-term Stress Skills include:

- Doing Mindful Meditation
- Spending time in nature
- Visualizing
- Drawing
- Writing in a journal
- Talking to a trusted friend or adult or therapist
- Helping someone else
- Any other actions that help you manage your stress

Different Stress Skills work for different people and for different situations. The Stress Skills that you use may be entirely different from those used by your friends, family, or classmates. It's important to try out numerous Stress Skills to find the ones that are most successful for you.

What short-term Stress Skills work for you when you are in your stress response?

- _____
- _____
- _____
- _____
- _____
- _____

What short-term Stress Skills do not work for you when you are in your stress response?

- _____
- _____
- _____
- _____
- _____
- _____

What long-term Stress Skills work best for managing your stress?

- _____
- _____
- _____
- _____
- _____
- _____

What long-term Stress Skills do not work for managing your stress?

- _____
- _____
- _____
- _____
- _____
- _____

Why are Stress Skills important for hope?

_____

_____

_____

_____

Short-Term Stress Skill Practice: Deep Breathing

Dr. Erwin Valencia provided an example of how to take deep breaths from your diaphragm. Spend the next 90 seconds practicing this deep breathing technique. How did you feel before taking the deep breaths? How did you feel after? Deep breathing is a great way to calm your mind, decrease your stress, and return to your upstairs brain.

_____

_____

_____

_____

Long-Term Stress Skill Practice: Journaling

When we have a lot to do, it can cause us to feel overwhelmed and activate our stress response. Sometimes the simple act of writing down all of the tasks we have on our minds helps to alleviate stress. It is especially helpful to do before we bed so that our mind is calm before we sleep. Take a few minutes to journal through your stressors.

Lesson 4 Inspired Action

Begin practicing Stress Skills when you find yourself in your downstairs brain or observe that you are experiencing your stress response. Try using Stress Skills that you don't typically use. Pay attention to how they affect your brain and biology.

Lesson 4 Friend Check in:

Did you check in with your Hopeful Mindsets friend today?   YES   NO

What did you discuss with them? Did they provide any interesting insights about this lesson?

_____

_____

What are their favorite Stress Skills for managing their stress response? Are they the same as yours? Different?

_____

_____

Do they have ways to identify their stress response that are different from your own?

_____

_____

HAPPINESS HABITS

Happiness Habits are healthy, long-term actions that cause your brain to release happiness hormones including endorphins, dopamine, serotonin, and oxytocin. Happiness Habits help you stay in your upstairs brain, where you access the problem-solving skills, collaboration, and passion critical for hope.

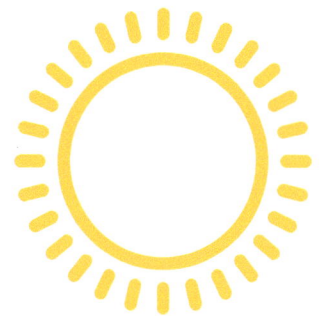

Positive Feelings

Positive feelings, the first ingredient of hope, are feelings that are located in your upstairs brain like wonder, joy, and peace that make it easier to overcome obstacles that get in the way of hope. You proactively manage the emotional despair of hopelessness using Stress Skills and use your Happiness Habits to stay in your upstairs brain, where you then energetically move towards your goals in life.

Activating purpose	Exercising / Nutrition	Volunteering
Pursuing passion	Creating / listening to music	Wonder/Awe
Utilizing strengths		Quality sleep
	Dancing / Singing	Doodling
Meditation	Drawing / Painting	
Smiling	Gratitude	

Read the Lesson 5 text and watch the Lesson 5 Hopeful Mindsets course videos, then answer the questions below:

The Second Key to Shine Hope

The Second Key to Shine Hope is fostering Habits for Happiness. Happiness Habits are healthy, long-term actions that cause your brain to release happiness hormones including endorphins, dopamine, serotonin, and oxytocin. Happiness Habits help you stay in your upstairs brain, where you access the problem-solving skills, collaboration, and passion critical for hope.

Some examples of short-term Stress Skills include:

- Utilizing strengths
- Pursuing passion
- Activating purpose
- Smiling
- Exercising/Nutrition
- Playing or Listening to Music
- Spending Time in Nature
- Showing Gratitude and Kindness
- Playing Games
- Volunteering

- Time with Family and Friends
- Experiencing Wonder & Awe
- Practicing Faith
- Sleeping
- Dancing and Singing
- Donating
- Giving a hug
- Setting Goals
- Practicing Affirmations

How are Happiness Habits different than Stress Skills?

_____

_____

Why are Happiness Habits important for hope?

_____

_____

When we get busy or stressed, we tend to skip our Happiness Habits. However, these are the times when we need Happiness Habits most, as they help us maintain our hopeful mindset. What are the "non-negotiable" Happiness Habits that you make time for in your daily or weekly schedule?

_____

_____

_____

_____

Who can you practice your Happiness Habits with?

_____

_____

Practicing Happiness Habits: Gratitude

This exercise is an excerpt from Dr. Dan Tomasulo's book, "Learned Hopefulness." Take five minutes to write down everything that happened yesterday. Pay attention to what happened, how it made you feel, and how you responded. Focus on your thoughts and feelings during your reflection.

Gratitude is one of the Happiness Habits that can help us stay in our upstairs brain. Take the next five minutes to once again write down everything that happened yesterday, but now, frame it through the lens of gratitude. What were you grateful for? When things didn't go as you wanted or you were emotionally triggered, what could you find to still be grateful for?

How did the day change based on your lens? How can you start incorporating this practice more regularly?

Making Time for Happiness Habits

Take time to practice at least one new Happiness Habit each day this week.

What Happiness Habits did you practice this week?

1. _____   5. _____

2. _____   6. _____

3. _____   7. _____

4. _____

Which Happiness Habits did you enjoy the most?

_____

_____

Think about the Happiness Habit you enjoyed the most, and answer the following questions:

How did your body feel before practicing your Happiness Habit?

_____

_____

How did your body feel during your Happiness Habit?

_____

_____

How did your body feel after practicing your Happiness Habit?

_____

_____

How did the Happiness Habit impact your beliefs? Thoughts?

_____

_____

Lesson 5 Inspired Action

Take time to do at least one Happiness Habit each day. Pay attention to how you feel before, during, and after your Happiness Habits. Like your Stress Skills, everyone has different Happiness Habits. It's important to remember that you might have to try a few before you find the one that works for you. Keep track of your Happiness Habits in the "Making Time for Happiness Habits" section above.

Lesson 5 Friend Check in:

Did you check in with your Hopeful   YES   NO
Mindsets friend today?

What did you discuss with them? Did they provide any interesting insights about this lesson?

_____

_____

What Happiness Habits do they practice regularly? Have you tried their Happiness Habits before?

_____

_____

How do they feel before doing their Happiness Habits? How do they feel after?

_____

_____

What did each of you identify as non-negotiable Happiness Habits?

_____

_____

INSPIRED ACTIONS

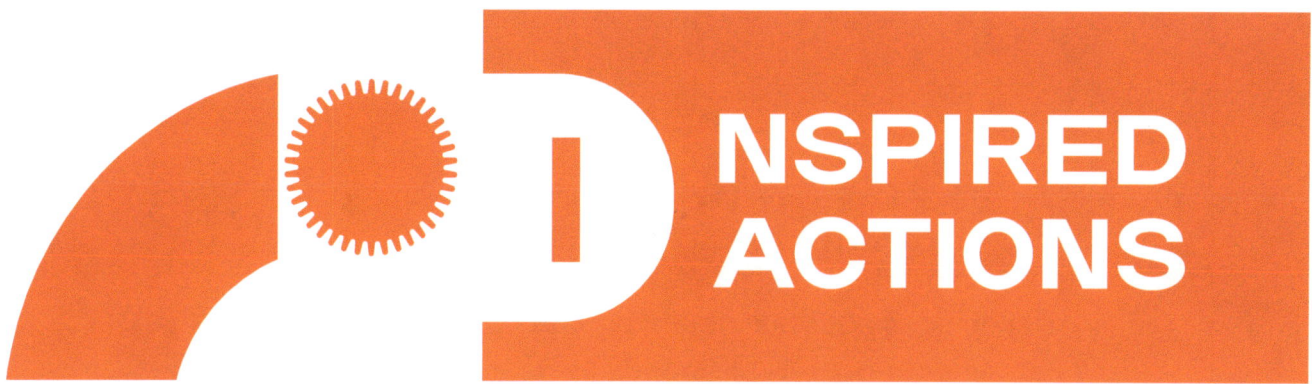

Inspired Actions, the second ingredient of hope, are the deliberate steps you take toward your goals in life. Inspired Actions help you to move away from the motivational helplessness, the second ingredient of hopelessness, and toward what you are hopeful for in life.

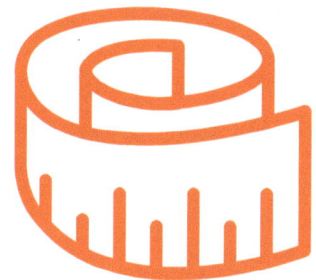

Types of Goals:

WOOP

Achievement

Intrinsic

SMART

Stretch

Micro-Goals

Pathways, Agency, and Regoaling

Obstacles are inevitable, and sometimes you can't reach the goal as you intended. It is important to embrace obstacles to goals, learn to pivot or reevaluate, be flexible and adaptable, and never be afraid to ask for help.

If a goal seems too big, use the stepping process or create micro-goals to chunk it down into smaller goals. Think of one thing you can do in the next 20 minutes. And know when you need to re-goal.

S.M.A.R.T. Goals

SPECIFIC

Be specific about your goal. Think about these questions when creating your goal: What needs to be accomplished? Who is responsible for it? What steps will you take to achieve it?

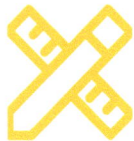

MEASURABLE

Can you measure your progress? If this goal will take a long time to achieve, set shorter term goals to reach along the way.

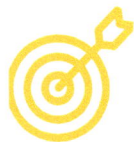

ACHIEVABLE

Are you inspired and motivated to reach your goal? Do you have the tools or skills you need? If not, do you know how you can get them?

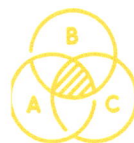

RELEVANT

Does your goal make sense? Does it go along with what you are trying to achieve in the bigger picture?

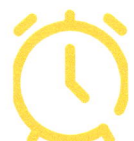

TIME-BOUND

Is your timing realistic? Can you achieve your goal in the time period set? Think about what you may want to achieve at the halfway point.

Lesson 6: **INSPIRED ACTIONS**
COURSE REFLECTION

Read the Lesson 6 text and watch the Lesson 6 Hopeful Mindsets course videos, then answer the questions below:

Strengths, Passion, and Purpose

Write down the top five strengths identified in the VIA Character Strengths Survey that you completed during Preparation Day:

1. _____

2. _____

3. _____

4. _____

5. _____

Brainstorm some things you are currently passionate about:

_____

_____

Based on your list above, brainstorm how to use your strengths to fulfill your passions and find your purpose. Write down ideas or use drawings or maps to organize your thoughts:

What career paths might you pursue to fulfill this purpose?

_____

_____

_____

_____

> **Remember:** You will likely have multiple passions and throughout your life, and your strengths will continue to grow and change. It is therefore important to periodically re-examine your passions and strengths to ensure you are continuing to take inspired actions towards fulfilling your purpose.

The Third Key to Shine Hope

The Third Key to Shine Hope is taking Inspired Actions using a variety of goal-setting techniques. To ensure your goals are helping you foster hope, we recommend using the six frameworks and types of goals discussed in this lesson:

ACHIEVEMENT GOALS: Achievement goals are those aimed at accomplishing an outcome (i.e. being on time), rather than avoiding a mistake or failure (i.e. not being late). We want all the goals we set to be achievement, rather than avoidant, in nature.

INTRINSIC GOALS: Intrinsic goals are goals that pertain to your passions and core values, and are always focused on one of three things: meaningful relationships, personal growth, or community contributions. Extrinsic goals, by comparison, are goals that focus on achieving something outside of yourself, such as obtaining power or the approval of others.

THE WOOP FRAMEWORK: WOOP helps you brainstorm goals by writing down your Wish, Outcome, Obstacle, and Plan. It is a general way to think about a framework for goals and is important to use for goals related to health, community, education, relationships, work, and more.

SMART GOALS: This is a framework to build on WOOP. It's important that each goal we set, whether it be a big goal or a small goal, is Specific, Measureable, Achievable, Relevant, and Time-bound. This gives us clarity, focus, and accountability, and ensures we set goals that are relevant to us and what we are passionate about in life.

STRETCH GOALS: Stretch goals are those that push our limits, challenge us to think bigger and broader, and take us beyond SMART. They are inspirational and aspirational, and we want to add these to stretch us. Having several long-term goals that challenge you to grow keeps you focused on the future.

MICRO-GOALS: Micro-goals are the small, achievable goals that help you move toward your stretch goals. They are the steps in the stepping process that help you continue looking towards the future.

Read about each of these techniques in Lesson 6, then answer the prompts below.

Why are goals important for hope?

_____

_____

Think about a goal you currently have for yourself. Is it an achievement or avoidance goal? An intrinsic or extrinsic goal? If it is an avoidance or extrinsic goal, how can you rework the goal to ensure it is an achievement and intrinsic goal?

_____

_____

Why is it important to set both stretch goals and micro-goals?

_____

_____

Goal-Setting with Hope

When you are setting goals, remember that you are more than just your college classes or your future career. It's important to set goals not just in your professional life, but also in the other areas of your life that are important to you.

For each of the following areas of your life, follow the goal-setting prompts below: College, relationships or personal life, health and well-being, hope, community.

Goal for College

Using the WOOP method, brainstorm a goal you want to achieve:

Wish: _____

Outcome: _____

Obstacle: _____

Plan: _____

Take your "plan" above and turn it into a stretch goal.

Stretch Goal:

_____

_____

Is your Stretch Goal:

An achievement goal?   YES   NO

An intrinsic goal?   YES   NO

If you answered no to either of the questions above, try to think of a new stretch goal.

Goal for College *(con't)*

Set three micro-goals that will help you take inspired actions toward your stretch goal:

1._____

2._____

3._____

Confirm that your micro-goals are SMART goals:

Are they:	HOW?
SPECIFIC	_____
MEASURABLE	_____
ACHIEVABLE	_____
RELEVANT	_____
TIME-BOUND	_____

Goal for Relationships or Personal Life

Using the WOOP method, brainstorm a goal you want to achieve:

Wish: _____

Outcome: _____

Obstacle: _____

Plan: _____

Take your "plan" above and turn it into a stretch goal.

Goal for Relationships or Personal Life *(con't)*

Stretch Goal:

_____

_____

Is your Stretch Goal:

An achievement goal?	YES	NO
An intrinsic goal?	YES	NO

If you answered no to either of the questions above, try to think of a new stretch goal.

Set three micro-goals that will help you take inspired actions toward your stretch goal:

1._____

2._____

3._____

Confirm that your micro-goals are SMART goals:

Are they: HOW?

SPECIFIC   _____

MEASURABLE   _____

ACHIEVABLE   _____

RELEVANT   _____

TIME-BOUND   _____

Goal for Health and Well-being

Using the WOOP method, brainstorm a goal you want to achieve:

Wish: _____

Outcome: _____

Obstacle: _____

Plan: _____

Take your "plan" above and turn it into a stretch goal.

Stretch Goal:

_____

_____

Is your Stretch Goal:

An achievement goal?   YES   NO

An intrinsic goal?   YES   NO

If you answered no to either of the questions above, try to think of a new stretch goal.

Set three micro-goals that will help you take inspired actions toward your stretch goal:

1. _____

2. _____

3. _____

Goal for Health and Well-being *(con't)*

Confirm that your micro-goals are SMART goals:

Are they: **HOW?**

    SPECIFIC   _____

    MEASURABLE   _____

    ACHIEVABLE   _____

    RELEVANT   _____

    TIME-BOUND   _____

Goal for Hope

Using the WOOP method, brainstorm a goal you want to achieve:

Wish: _____

Outcome: _____

Obstacle: _____

Plan: _____

Take your "plan" above and turn it into a stretch goal.

Stretch Goal:

_____

_____

Is your Stretch Goal:

An achievement goal?   YES   NO

An intrinsic goal?   YES   NO

If you answered no to either of the questions above, try to think of a new stretch goal.

Goal for Hope *(con't)*

Set three micro-goals that will help you take inspired actions toward your stretch goal:

1. _____

2. _____

3. _____

Confirm that your micro-goals are SMART goals:

Are they: **HOW?**

SPECIFIC _____

MEASURABLE _____

ACHIEVABLE _____

RELEVANT _____

TIME-BOUND _____

Goal for my Community

Using the WOOP method, brainstorm a goal you want to achieve:

Wish: _____

Outcome: _____

Obstacle: _____

Plan: _____

Take your "plan" above and turn it into a stretch goal.

Goal for my Community *(con't)*

Stretch Goal:

_____

_____

Is your Stretch Goal:

An achievement goal?   YES   NO

An intrinsic goal?   YES   NO

If you answered no to either of the questions above, try to think of a new stretch goal.

Set three micro-goals that will help you take inspired actions toward your stretch goal:

1._____

2._____

3._____

Confirm that your micro-goals are SMART goals:

Are they: **HOW?**

SPECIFIC   _____

MEASURABLE   _____

ACHIEVABLE   _____

RELEVANT   _____

TIME-BOUND   _____

Lesson 6 Inspired Action

In his book *Learned Hopefulness*, Dr. Dan Tomasulo encourages you to set micro-goals by asking yourself, "what can I do in the next 20 minutes?" Each day this week, look at one of the stretch goals you set and brainstorm an inspired action you can take "in the next 20 minutes" to help you reach your goal.

Lesson 6 Friend Check in:

Did you check in with your Hopeful   YES   NO
Mindsets friend today?

What did you discuss with them? Did they provide any interesting insights about this lesson?

_____

_____

What stretch goals did they set? Are they similar to yours or different?

_____

_____

If you are having a hard time discovering your passions, purpose, or goals, consider discussing them with your friend. After all, the people around us can sometimes identify things about us that we miss.

Read the Lesson 7 text and watch the Lesson 7 Hopeful Mindsets course videos, then answer the questions below:

Overcoming Obstacles

Write down each of your goals from Lesson 6, as well as the limiting beliefs, affirming beliefs, potential obstacles, and solutions that are associated with each one:

Stretch Goal for College:

_____

_____

Limiting belief I have: _____

Reaffirming belief I will replace it with: _____

Potential obstacles I might face:

    1. _____

    2. _____

Solutions I can use to overcome these obstacles:

    1. _____

    2. _____

One person I can check in with as it relates to this goal:

_____

Stretch Goal for Relationships or Personal Life:

_____

_____

Limiting belief I have: _____

Reaffirming belief I will replace it with: _____

Potential obstacles I might face:

1. _____

2. _____

Solutions I can use to overcome these obstacles:

1. _____

2. _____

One person I can check in with as it relates to this goal:

_____

Stretch Goal for Health and Well-being:

_____

_____

Limiting belief I have: _____

Reaffirming belief I will replace it with: _____

Potential obstacles I might face:

1. _____

2. _____

Stretch Goal for Health and Well-being: *(con't)*

Solutions I can use to overcome these obstacles:

1. _____

2. _____

One person I can check in with as it relates to this goal:

_____

Stretch Goal for Hope:

_____

_____

Limiting belief I have: _____

Reaffirming belief I will replace it with: _____

Potential obstacles I might face:

1. _____

2. _____

Solutions I can use to overcome these obstacles:

1. _____

2. _____

One person I can check in with as it relates to this goal:

_____

Stretch Goal for Community:

_____

_____

Limiting belief I have: _____

Reaffirming belief I will replace it with: _____

Potential obstacles I might face:

    1. _____

    2. _____

Solutions I can use to overcome these obstacles:

    1. _____

    2. _____

One person I can check in with as it relates to this goal:

_____

Sometimes we run into obstacles that cannot be overcome, and we have to reexamine our goal. When might we need to regoal? When is a time that you have had to regoal in the past?

_____

_____

_____

_____

Why is it important to not be attached to your stretch goals?

_____

_____

Lesson 7 Inspired Action

Using the visualization audio guide in your Lesson, choose one of the stretch goals you set in Lesson 6 and visualize reaching your goal for five minutes. How did you accomplish your goal? What specific steps did you have to take or obstacles did you have to overcome? How did you overcome the obstacles? How did you feel when you accomplished it? Repeat this process with each of your remaining goals.

Lesson 7 Friend Check in:

Did you check in with your Hopeful   YES   NO
Mindsets friend today?

What did you discuss with them? Did they provide any interesting insights about this lesson?

_____

_____

Discuss the obstacles that each of you might face when striving to achieve your goals. Was your friend able to identify different obstacles that you hadn't previously considered?

_____

_____

Help each other identify solutions to the potential obstacles to your goals. Were they able to identify more solutions to your potential obstacles?

_____

_____

Identify a time to check in with each other on your goal status. Write down the date and time here:

_____

_____

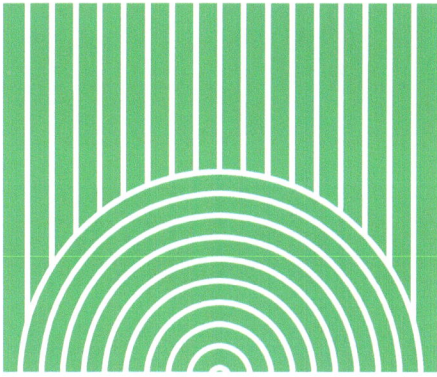

NOURISHING NETWORKS

Your Nourishing Networks, also known as your Hope Networks, are the people in your life that provide you with support, help you stay on track, encourage you to succeed, and who you do the same for in return. You are up to 95% more likely to achieve a goal if you write it down, and check in with someone regularly. So Nourishing Networks are critical support systems for moving you towards what you hope for in life.

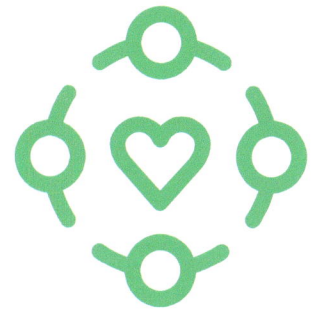

Your Hope Networks should include:

People who know and understand you.

People who value your strengths.

People who activate the SHINE framework.

People whom you trust and can confide in.

People who are available to support you.

People you are willing to do the above for as well.

Enhancing Your Hope Networks

Enhance your Hope Networks using the 5:1 rule, vulnerability, praise, recognition, kindness, gratitude, empathy, compassion, collaboration, and strong communication, and be sure to have different networks for different areas of life.

Don't forget to include doctors, therapists, and/or other medical professionals in your Hope Networks.

Lesson 8: **NETWORK FOR HOPE**
COURSE REFLECTION

Read the Lesson 8 text and watch the Lesson 8 Hopeful Mindsets course videos, then answer the questions below:

Identifying Your Social Connections

Use the blank space on the next page to create your network of social connections. Choose a symbol for yourself, place yourself anywhere on the sheet, and put your first name in the middle of the symbol.

Draw everyone in your life now, with individual symbols or shapes, and place them as close to or far away from you, as large or as small, as you want. These can be positive or negative relationships. There are no right or wrong ways to do this.

Of the people you have drawn in your social connection web, identify one person with whom you'd be willing to increase your connection. Think about the various ways to do this and pick one. Could it be a text, a call, or a visit? Might you send an email or card? Find one way to extend your contact. Deepening our present connections is a good way to enhance well-being.

Having more hope in your life not only means more contact and connection with those that we have a positive association with already; it also means reducing the connection with people who drag our energy down and drain us. Go back and look at your social connection web again. Who has a negative influence on you? What could you do to reduce the contact you have with them?

As you continue through this course, consider coming back and updating this web as you make new friends or alter your connections with the people already represented.

"You are the average of the five people you spend the most time with."
Who are the five people you spend the most time with? Do they support you, accept you, and help you to reach your goals?

1. _____

2. _____

3. _____

4. _____

5. _____

The Fourth Key to Shine Hope

The Fourth Key to Shine Hope is your Nourishing Networks. Your Nourishing Networks, also known as your Hope Networks, are the people in your life that provide you with support, help you stay on track, encourage you to succeed, and who you do the same for in return.

Once you've drawn your social connections, begin to brainstorm the people who belong in your Hope Network:

Friends and Family I count on:

People I turn to for Stress Skills:

People I practice Happy Habits with:

Things I can connect to: *ex. Spiritual Advisor, Peer Support, Colleagues, Pets, Nature*

Medical experts I can turn to when I need help:

Campus resources I can utilize:

Check our list of resources for additional info
ex. If you can't list anyone, you can check out our list of resources for how to get connected.

SCAN FOR OTHER RESOURCES

Creating Hope Networks for Your Goals

When we set goals, it is important to create a Hope Network of people who will support us and help us reach our goals. Your Hope Network might be slightly different for each goal you set, as different people can help us with different things. Take time to reflect on who in your Hope Network can help you to achieve each of your goals from Lesson 6:

Stretch Goal for College:

_____

_____

People in your Hope Network for this goal:

_____

_____

Stretch Goal for relationships or personal life:

_____

_____

People in your Hope Network for this goal:

_____

_____

Stretch Goal for health and well-being:

_____

_____

People in your Hope Network for this goal:

_____

_____

Stretch Goal for hope:

_____

_____

People in your Hope Network for this goal:

_____

_____

Stretch Goal for community:

_____

_____

People in your Hope Network for this goal:

_____

_____

Now that you've identified people in your Hope Network, how can you strengthen it? The 5:1 rule states that for every one negative or constructive criticism you say to someone, you should say five positive things. Pick one person from your Hope Networks and write down five things you love about them. Once you've written down all five, call or text the person you chose and tell them all five things

1 _____

2 _____

3 _____

4 _____

5 _____

Remember, the size of your Hope Network doesn't matter, the quality of your connections matters. The best way to receive support is to give support.

Lesson 8 Inspired Action

Take time to strengthen your Hope Network. Each day this week, use one of the techniques for enhancing your Hope Network (5:1 rule, vulnerability, praise, recognition, kindness, gratitude, empathy, and compassion, forgiveness, and self-forgiveness).

Bonus Action: Focus on your interactions throughout the week. Try to follow the 5:1 Rule with everyone you speak to. Take notes on whether or not you are successful.

Lesson 8 Friend Check in:

Did you check in with your Hopeful   YES   NO
Mindsets friend today?

What did you discuss with them? Did they provide any interesting insights about this lesson?

_____

_____

Compare your social connection circles. How were they the same? How were they different?

_____

_____

Practice the 5:1 rule with your friend! Write down five nice things about them here and then exchange your answers.

_____

_____

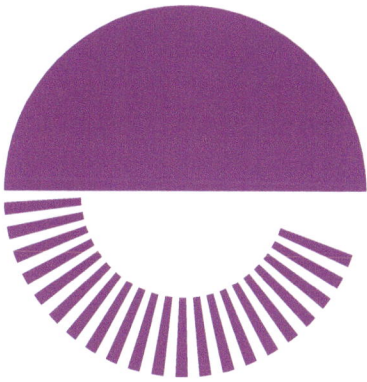

ELIMINATING CHALLENGES

Challenges to Hope are negative habits of thought that quickly take you to hopelessness, that emotional despair and sense of helplessness. The thought patterns are often unconscious habits, so becoming aware of these patterns is critical. Once we know what they are and recognize them, it is important to counteract them so that we don't let them keep us from all we hope for in life.

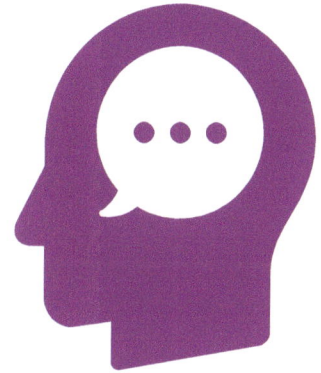

Eliminating Challenges

Most of the Challenges to Hope take constant, repetitive actions to change and overcome. Thanks to the science of neuroplasticity, we know it is possible with practice and dedication. The key is to learn to identify what specific challenges happen most frequently and then proactively find ways to manage those challenges.

Limiting beliefs	Focusing on Uncontrollables	Mind Wandering
Automatic Negative Thoughts (ANTs)	Attaching to outcomes	Implicity Bias
All-or-nothing thinking	Internalizing failure	Negative Framing
Negative bias	Toxic Consumption	Perfectionism
Rumination & Worry	Nocebo Effect	Taking things personally

Read the Lesson 9 text and watch the Lesson 9 Hopeful Mindsets course videos, then answer the questions below:

The Fifth Key to Shine Hope

The Fifth Key to Shine Hope is Eliminating the Challenges to Hope. Challenges to Hope are negative habits of thought that quickly take you to hopelessness, that emotional despair and sense of helplessness. The thought patterns are often unconscious habits we don't realize we're doing, so becoming aware of these patterns is critical. Once we know what they are and recognize them, it is important to counteract them so that we don't let them keep us from all we hope for in life.

Go through each challenge and reflect on when you have encountered the challenges to hope, how you have overcome them in the past, and how you can overcome them even more successfully in the future.

Challenge #1: Limiting Beliefs

Have you noticed any recurring limiting beliefs you've had since you've started this course? _____

What is one limiting belief you have about yourself, hope, or college?

_____

_____

Ask yourself Byron Katie's four questions about your limiting belief:

1 Is it true? _____

2 Can you absolutely know that it's true? _____

3 How do you react when you believe that thought?

_____

Challenge #1: Limiting Beliefs *(con't)*

4 Who would you be without that thought?

_____

What is a reaffirming belief you can use instead?

_____

Challenge #2: Automatic Negative Thoughts

What is one ANT you've had in the last week?

_____

_____

How did you respond to the ANT?

_____

_____

What Stress Skills and reaffirming beliefs could you use to respond even better in the future?

_____

_____

Challenge #3: All-or-Nothing Thinking

When is one time that you have used all-or-nothing thinking in the past?

_____

_____

How can you reframe your thoughts to avoid all-or-nothing thinking in the future?

_____

_____

When you find yourself using all-or-nothing thinking, what is one Stress Skill that you can use to return to your upstairs brain?

_____

_____

Challenge #4: Negative Bias

Reflect on the last day. Was there a time that something negative drew your attention away from something positive?

_____

_____

What Stress Skills or Happiness Habits could you use to counteract negative bias?

_____

_____

Challenge #5: Rumination

What is one thing you found yourself ruminating about today?

_____

_____

What Stress Skill did you use (or could you use) to break the rumination cycle and return to your upstairs brain?

_____

_____

What Happiness Habit did you use (or could you use) to stay in your upstairs brain?

_____

_____

Challenge #6: Worry

What is one thing you found yourself worrying about today?

_____

_____

Challenge #6: Worry *(con't)*

What Stress Skill did you use (or you could use) to break the worry cycle and return to your upstairs brain?

_____

_____

What Happiness Habit did you use (or you could use) to stay in your upstairs brain?

_____

_____

Challenge #7: Focusing on Uncontrollables

Focusing on things we cannot control can force us into rumination and worry cycles.

What Stress Skills can you use to release the worry and stress from the things you cannot control?

_____

_____

What Stress Skills can you take to release the worry from the things you CAN control?

_____

_____

In the sunflower below, write down the things you can control. In the areas around the sunflower, write down the things you cannot control. It's important to focus on things inside the sunflower and find ways to release the stress and worry associated with the things outside of the sunflower.

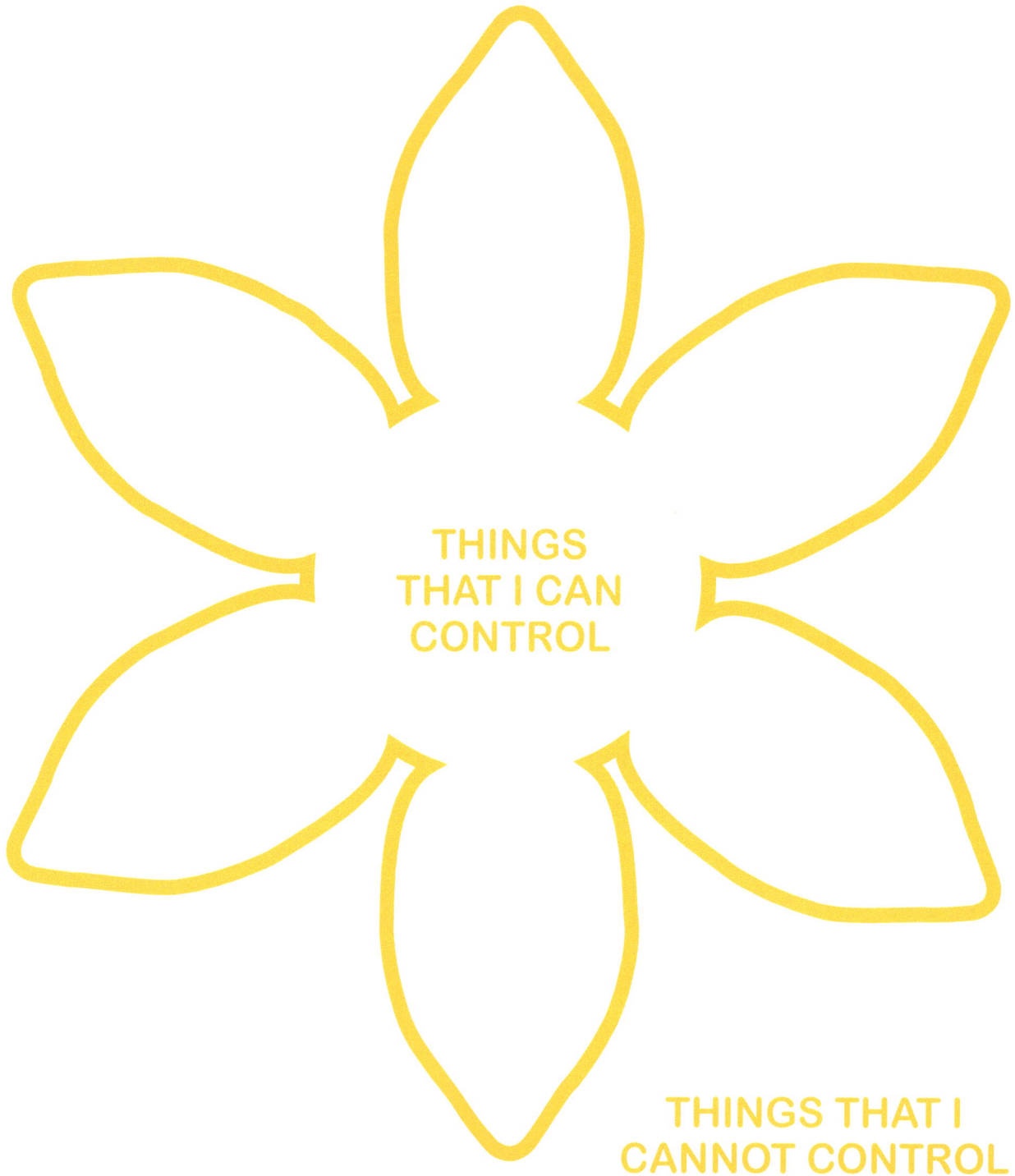

THINGS
THAT I CAN
CONTROL

THINGS THAT I
CANNOT CONTROL

Challenge #7: Focusing on Uncontrollables *(con't)*

Are there inspired actions you can take to solve the things within your control? What are they?

_____

_____

_____

_____

Challenge #8: Attaching to Outcomes

Have you put an unhealthy attachment on a goal or outcome in the past?

_____

_____

Did you reach that goal? If not, how did it feel when you were unable to obtain the outcome you wanted?

_____

_____

What did you want to feel by achieving that goal? What other goal can you set to help you achieve those same feelings?

_____

_____

Challenge #9: Internalizing Failure

Think of a time when you experienced failure. What step in the process failed?

_____

_____

Did you internalize the failure?

_____

_____

Challenge #9: Internalizing Failure *(con't)*

Why did the step in the process fail?

_____

_____

What can you do to prevent the same failure in the future?

_____

_____

What can you do to break this pattern of internalizing failure?

_____

_____

How do these challenges impact hope and your ability to reach your goals?

_____

_____

_____

_____

What strengths can you use to overcome the challenges to hope?

_____

_____

Which challenge to hope do you find the most difficult to overcome and why?

_____

_____

Lesson 9 Inspired Action

Pay attention when you encounter challenges to hope. When you feel yourself beginning to enter a rumination or worry cycle, attach to outcomes, internalize failure, or focus on the uncontrollables, take a 90-second pause and use your favorite Stress Skill to return to the present moment and your upstairs brain. Continue to practice replacing limiting beliefs, ANTs, and negative biases with reaffirming beliefs and a hopeful mindset.

Lesson 9 Friend Check in:

Did you check in with your Hopeful   YES   NO
Mindsets friend today?

What did you discuss with them? Did they provide any interesting insights about this lesson?

_____

_____

What is one challenge to hope that they have faced recently? How did they overcome it? Were there other ways they could have overcome the challenge to hope?

_____

_____

What is one challenge they have the hardest time overcoming? Share strategies.

_____

_____

Lesson 10: CREATING A VISION FOR YOUR FUTURE USING HOPE
COURSE REFLECTION

Read the Lesson 10 text and watch the Lesson 10 Hopeful Mindsets course videos, then answer the questions below:

Measuring Your Hope

Now that you have reached the end of the course, take a moment to retake the Snyder Hope Scale to find your new Hope Score.

Use the link provided to take the Snyder Hope Scale Assessment:
www.hopefulmindsets.com/hope-scales/

My initial Snyder Hope Scale Score: _____ /64

My Current Snyder Hope Scale Score: _____ /64

Did your score increase or decrease?

_____

_____

What positively or negatively impacted your score?

_____

_____

Remember, your hope score will rise and fall as you go throughout your life. The score is simply a way for you to check in with yourself and keep yourself centered and focused on your hope journey.

Activating Hope on Campus

What are some ways that you can help activate hope on your college campus?

_____

_____

_____

_____

How can you use the hope skills you have learned to share hope with others in your community?

_____

_____

_____

_____

Hopeful Mindsets Course Reflection

Your hope journey doesn't end at the end of this course. Just like any skill you want to improve, you must continue to practice your hope skills each and every day. As you reflect on your hope journey, consider what you've learned over the last 10 weeks and how you will continue to inspire hope both in your own life, and in the lives of those around you:

What Stress Skills have worked for you?

_____

_____

_____

_____

What Happiness Habits do you love doing?

_____
_____
_____
_____

What goals have you set or achieved over the last 10 weeks? (Remember, finishing this course is a goal, and one that you have now completed!)

_____
_____
_____
_____

What obstacles have you overcome?

_____
_____
_____
_____

How has your understanding of hope changed since the beginning of this course?

_____
_____
_____
_____

Why is hope a critical part of your life?

_____
_____
_____
_____

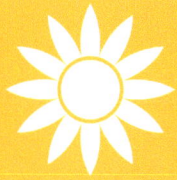

☀ MY HOPE HERO

HOW HOPEFUL ARE YOU?

Did you measure your hope? The lower your score, the more you want to practice these skills! Remember, hope is a muscle we need to build it (add it).

Check out here to get your hope score.

To write your hope hero journey, spend 20% of your time writing about their challenge, and 80% of the time sharing strategies for how they overcame it so others can learn from it. Here's how:

1. Write your hope hero's name in the yellow line next to the box (feel free to use a nickname or anything else).

2. Put your favorite photo of them on the yellow box, or an image of something that represents your hope hero.

3. Write an introduction explaining the challenge they faced. Explain the two ingredients of hopelessness: despair (feelings) and helplessness (inability to act) they experienced.

4. Share sadness, anger, fear, or other feelings, and choose 3 **Stress Skills** they used to navigate them (from the Shine infographic, or choose your own!).

5. Share 3 **Happiness Habits** they used to get back to upstairs brain.

6. Talk about 3 **Inspired Actions** they took, or share how your hope hero chunked down goals, the types of goals they've set, or if they had to regoal.

7. Share who was in their **Nourishing Network**, and how it helped them navigate the challenge.

8. Pick 3 challenges from the **'Eliminating Challenges'** on the infographic, and share how your hope hero eliminated them.

9. Write the conclusion. What do you want the world to know? What do you wish someone had told you? What is the moral of the story?

If you're inspired, share this hope hero story so we can help activate these skills globally!

#Hope #ShineHope #MyHopeHero

We all experience moments of hopelessness (emotional despair and motivational helplessness). The key is to use the Shine Hope skills to navigate your way from despair to positive feelings, and helplessness to inspired actions. Use the Shine Hope framework to build your muscle.

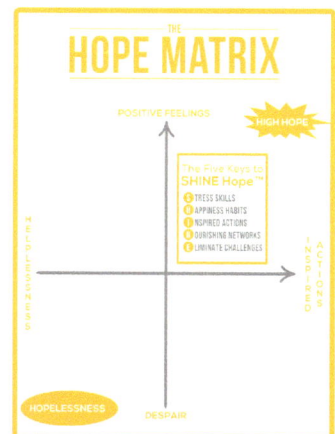

THE **HOPE MATRIX**

POSITIVE FEELINGS

HIGH HOPE

The Five Keys to
SHINE Hope
- STRESS SKILLS
- HAPPINESS HABITS
- INSPIRED ACTIONS
- NOURISHING NETWORKS
- ELIMINATE CHALLENGES

HOPELESSNESS

DESPAIR

MY HOPE HERO

To add image in this area, edit the PDF via Adobe Acrobat or any PDF app editor.

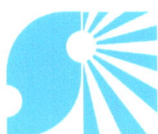

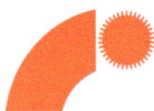

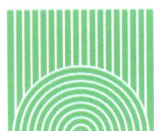

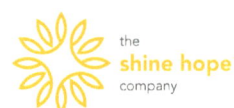

MY HOPE HERO

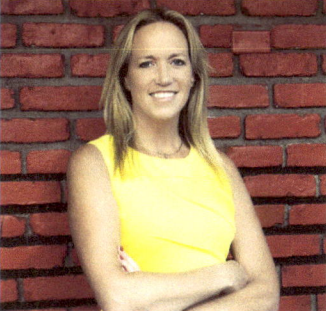

☀ Kathryn Goetzke

When Kathryn was 18 years old, a freshman at the University of Iowa, her dad died by suicide. It really changed her life. When she was in her early 20's, she then tried to take her own life, yet didn't tell another soul for 10 years. She knows a lot about hopelessness.

To work on her recovery, she used a lot of Stress Skills. She talks about crying, going to therapy, learning to meditate, deep breathing, and listening to music. She traveled a lot, and took up hiking and exercise. She also took up boxing and spent a lot of time in nature.

Kathryn was diligent about her Happiness Habits. She listened to her favorite band the Killers, went to concerts, focused on her nutrition and sleep, and started exercising. She pursued her passions, started a nonprofit iFred, and did a lot of volunteer work. She got serious about her purpose.

Kathryn also took a lot of Inspired Actions towards her goals. She chunked them down, got a degree and then an MBA. She couldn't talk to her dad anymore, so she found business mentors. Her brothers were always there to support her, and her mom was a source of strength and inspiration.

Kathryn spent a lot of time with her Nourishing Networks. She spent time with people that were kind, compassionate, fun, and helped her heal. She had a therapist and got close to God. She had animals and spent a lot of time with wild horses in Nevada.

She worked to Eliminate Challenges like her rumination and worry. She learned about sensory engagement, and even started a company to teach others. She worked to forgive herself and others. She focused on what she could control, which was her present and future, and did her best to let go of the rest. She put all her failures into teaching others.

Her use of the Shine Hope framework led her on a much healthier path. She has been sober almost 20 years, and had her nonprofit that same amount of time. She is a representative at the United Nations for the World Federation for Mental Health, and has shared her story around the world at places like the World Bank, Harvard, the United Nations, and more. She has created programming to teach hope to kids, published papers, and is now doing workplace programming, has a college, course, and is activating cities. She is on a mission to ensure all know how to hope, one person at a time. She is an inspiration, and someone that truly lives by example practicing all she teaches.

#Hope #ShineHope #MyHopeHero

the
shine hope
company

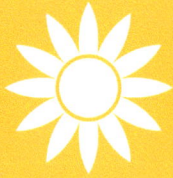

MY SHINE HOPE STORY™

HOW HOPEFUL ARE YOU?

Did you measure your hope? The lower your score, the more you want to practice these skills! Remember, hope is a muscle we need to build it (add it).

Check out here to get your hope score.

To write your own shine hope story, spend 20% of your time writing about your challenge, and 80% of the time sharing strategies for how you overcame it so others can learn from you. Here's how:

1. Write your name in the yellow line next to the box (feel free to use a nickname or anything else).

2. Put your favorite photo on the yellow box, or an image of something that represents you.

3. Write an introduction to your story explaining the challenge you faced. Explain the two ingredients of hopelessness: despair (feelings) and helplessness (inability to act) you experienced.

4. Share sadness, anger, fear, or other feelings, and choose **3 Stress Skills** you used to naviate them (from the Shine infographic, or choose your own!).

5. Share **3 Happiness Habits** you used to get back to your upstairs brain.

6. Talk about **3 Inspired Actions** you took, or share how you chunked down goals, the types of goals you set, or if you had to regoal.

7. Share who was in your **Nourishing Network**, and how they helped you navigate the challenge.

8. Pick 3 challenges from the **'Eliminating Challenges'** on the infographic, and share how you eliminated them.

9. Write your conclusion. What do you want the world to know? What do you wish someone had told you? What is the moral of the story?

If you're inspired, share your story so we can help activate these skills globally.

#Hope #ShineHope #MyShineHopeStory

> We all experience moments of hopelessness (emotional despair and motivational helplessness). The key is to use the Shine Hope skills to navigate your way from despair to positive feelings, and helplessness to inspired actions. Use the Shine Hope framework to build your muscle.

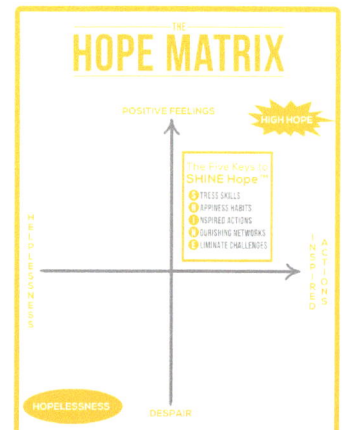

THE HOPE MATRIX

MY SHINE HOPE STORY™

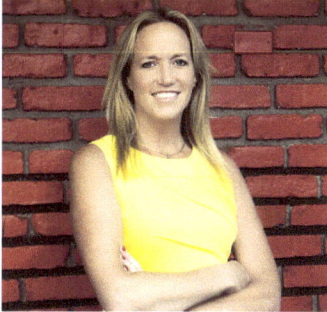

☀ Kathryn Goetzke

When I was 18 years old, a freshman at the University of Iowa, I called home and heard an unfamiliar, deep voice on the other line. It wasn't anyone I recognized, and he asked for my mom. My mom got on the phone to tell me my dad had taken his life. In that instance, my whole world crumbled. I felt a sadness so deep I thought I would never survive, and a helplessness so profound as I could not bring him back.

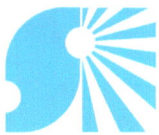

As hard as it was, I had to move forward. I started using Stress Skills to manage my pain. I cried when I was sad, started boxing to manage my anger, and learned how to start belly breathing to manage my fear. I listened to a lot of calming music when things got hard, and I started hiking all over the world. I also learned how to use sensory engagement to bring myself to the present moment.

Happiness Habits were critical. Sleep became an important part of my routine, and I started eating healthier foods. I cut alcohol out of my life. I replaced smoking with running, and made comedy clubs and laughter a part of my life. I listened to music, turned my sensory engagement passion into a purpose and started a company, and made volunteering a regular part of my life. I used dancing and live concerts (like my fave The Killers) as a form of release.

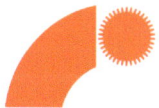

I also was very intentional about Inspired Actions. I had to chunk down my goals, leaving school and taking only one year at a time until I graduated. I had to regoal from having experiences with my dad to finding father-like figures to be in my life. I got closer to my brothers, their kids, and found mentors like Paul Carter and Dr. Belfer to guide me on my journey. My mom is my rock, my greatest source of strength and inspiration, keeping me moving forward towards my dreams.

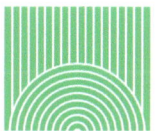

Nourishing Networks were a constant. I stayed close to my friends and family, traveling, dancing, studying, and laughing. They were so compassionate, kind, generous, fun, and helped me heal. I forgave my dad for leaving, and forgave myself for not being there for him when he needed me. I got very close to God, understanding that I couldn't save my dad, and that in time this lesson would teach me how to help others.

It wasn't easy to Eliminate Challenges like rumination, internalizing failure, or worry. Yet I studied sensory engagement to be present when my mind started running. I deconstructed what led to my dad taking his life in a way that made it clear how to save myself and others. I knew that I couldn't control my dad, just like I can't control others. So I have focused on creating programming yet not being attached to if people want to learn it.

It's not been the easiest journey, and takes work. Yet by using the Shine Hope framework I have created a new life that is full of wonder, awe, happiness, adventure, and meaning. A different one than I expected, yet a beautiful one because I was able to dive in my pain, and learn the lessons necessary to teach others. And I use all my dad taught me in business to create a Shine Hope model for the world that ensures all know the what, why, and how of hope. And for that I know he is so very proud.

No matter what life brings, Keep Shining.

#Hope #ShineHope #MyHopeStory

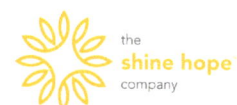

the shine hope company

MY SHINE HOPE STORY™

To add image in this area, edit the PDF via Adobe Acrobat or any PDF app editor.

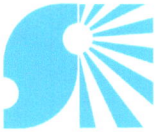

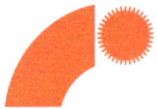

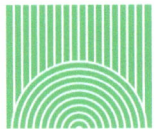

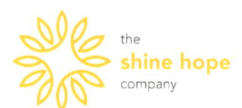

Lesson 10 Inspired Action

Hope is a lifelong journey. Take time to think about where you want your journey to go now that the course is coming to an end. What hope skills will you practice to continue to create, maintain, and grow your hope? How will you activate hope in the lives of those around you?

Lesson 10 Friend Check in:

Did you check in with your Hopeful   YES   NO
Mindsets friend today?

What did you discuss with them? Did they provide any interesting insights about this lesson?

_____

_____

Share your Hope Stories. Brainstorm how you can both make your hope stories reality:

_____

_____

Brainstorm additional hope initiatives that you could start at your university.

_____

_____

_____

_____

PLANT SUNFLOWER GARDENS TO SHINE HOPE

Gardening is a great time to practice the Shine Hope Framework, as we have a lot of challenges while planting a garden and we can go from hope to hopelessness pretty quickly. Yet that is a normal part of life, so gardening is an easy place to start practicing these skills.

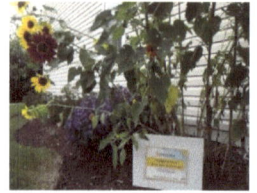

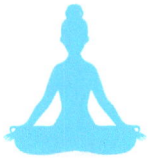

Say you find some tough ground you need to dig into to plant, you may get frustrated and give up. It is a good time to practice a **Stress Skill** like a 90-second pause or deep breathing, to calm down your stress response. Then try again! You may also notice when others get frustrated and teach them how to use this skill to navigate from their downstairs brain back upstairs.

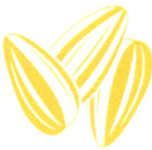

Eating the sunflower seeds (if ok with your doctor) might be a good way for you to practice your **Happiness Habits.** Sunflower seeds are nutritious, high in choline and selenium, great for brain function and memory. You might also get some exercise planting gardens, and spend time in nature, two other Happiness Habits and great ways to release endorphins.

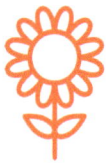

Planting gardens remind us to take **Inspired Actions** by setting specific goals for the garden. If we want a garden, we need to set a SMART goal about how many flowers, when and where we want the garden, and how we are going to grow the flowers. It is best if we write down the plan, chunk it down into actionable steps, think about obstacles and multiple ways we might overcome them, and check in with someone regularly to ensure progress.

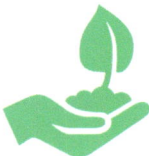

We can cultivate our **Nourishing Networks** by planting gardens with others. That way, if we have challenges while planting, we can face them together and be more creative about overcoming them. And if we don't live by the person we want to plant with, we can both decide to plant and check in regularly on the garden. It is also super fun to plan community gardens, or even fields of sunflowers, and all join together in learning and practicing skills to Shine Hope.

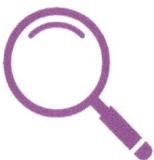

And finally, time to get serious about **Eliminating Challenges**. For example, if our sunflowers die and we fail for a season of planting, it is easy for us to think of ourselves as failures. Yet we aren't failures, our process failed. So deconstruct the process. Did we under or over water? Did we plant at the wrong time of year? Was something wrong with the soil? Did we overwater? It is time to investigate, and instead of ruminating about the sunflowers start figuring out what we can do better to try again next year.

Planting sunflowers is a way to spread the message of hope, as if you put up a Gardens of Hope sign with the website, people can then find the curriculum to learn more about the programs for 'how' to hope. Our program is available around the world, and gardens are a great way to share the message that Hope is Teachable.

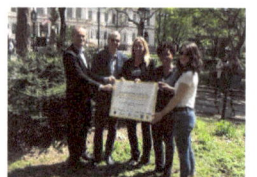

Find out more at

@theshinehopecompany

ADDITIONAL RESOURCES

Hopeful Minds is based on the research that hope is teachable. The aim is to equip all students, teachers, and parents with the tools they need to define, learn, and grow a Hopeful Mind. The Hopeful Minds curriculums and resources are available for download at www.hopefulminds.org/curriculums

The Five-Day Global Hope Challenge is a daily challenge that introduces the Five Keys to Shine Hope that everyone can use to activate hope within their lives and their community. The challenge is ideal for governments, workplaces, schools, and more. Sign-up today at www.hopefulcities.org

Friendship Bench's mission is to get people out of kufungisisa - depression & anxiety - by creating safe spaces and a sense of belonging in communities to improve mental wellbeing and enhance quality of life. To learn more and request a bench placed in your area, visit www.friendshipbenchzimbabwe.org

Karma Box Project is a community initiative allowing people to give non-perishable food, hygiene products, toiletries, and other useful items to those in need. The boxes are filled up with the goods by anyone in the community and someone in need can take items from the box as needed. To learn more, visit www.karmaboxproject.org

One World Strong Foundation created the ResilienceNet Mobile App, which empowers and provides support to local, regional, and national terrorism prevention practitioners, relevant frontline responders and individual Americans seeking support. To learn more about the One World Strong Foundation and download their app, visit www.oneworldstrong.org/copy-of-how-we-do-it

National Alliance on Mental Illness (NAMI) is America's largest grassroots mental health organization dedicated to building better lives for Americans affected by mental illness. NAMI offers an abundance of resources for those navigating mental illness or for those seeking to learn more. Find more at www.nami.org/home

Choose Love Movement nurtures safer and more loving communities through next generation essential life skills and character development programs for all stages of life. Choose Love is an evidence-based curriculum that will help students feel safer, learn better, and achieve more! Find out more at www.chooselovemovement.org

Hope Means Nevada works to eliminate teen suicide and empower Nevada's youth to live hopeful lives. Find out more at www.hopemeansnevada.org

One Mind catalyzes visionary change through science, business and media to transform the world's mental health. Find out more at www.onemind.org

Charter for Compassion supports the emerging global movement that brings compassion to life. It is a global network connecting people, cities, grassroots organizers and leaders to each other. It provides educational resources, organizing tools, and avenues for communication. Find out more at www.charterforcompassion.org

Hopeful Mindsets®

Hopeful Mindsets® is a framework that uses the Five Keys to Shine Hope to apply to any challenge in life. It is based on the work of leading experts on Hope, Mindset, Mental Health, Stress, Positive Psychology, Business, Communications, and more. Using the Five Keys to Shine Hope as a foundation, Hopeful Mindsets introduces critical hope skills to help anyone move from hopelessness to hope.

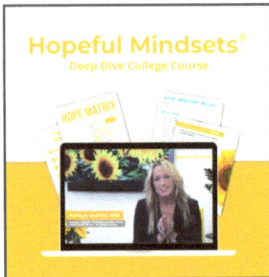

The initial program, Hopeful Mindsets on the College Campus, is a 10-module video course from The Shine Hope Company that equips students with crucial hope skills through expert insights and real-life stories. The course features experts from Harvard, Stanford, and Columbia, with insights from recent college graduates that offer real-life practical strategies and stories from their experiences with homelessness, mental health diagnoses, death, violence, and everyday challenges at school.

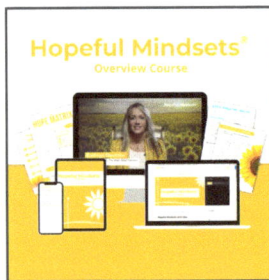

The Hopeful Mindsets General Overview is a 90-minute video course for anyone that introduces hope and the Five Keys to Shine Hope framework to help you create, maintain, and grow hope in your life. This course is taught by Kathryn Goetzke, based on her knowledge of mental health and hope, and her work to date. It compiles knowledge from leading experts on Hope, Mindset, Mental Health, Stress, Positive Psychology, Business, Communications, and includes video lessons, a full downloadable workbook and exercises to practice skills for hope, and is available individually or to license for organizations.

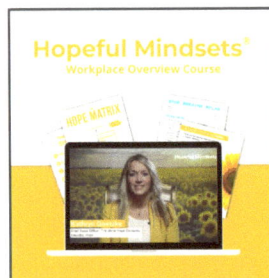

The Hopeful Mindsets Workplace Overview is a 90-minute video course for the workplace that introduces hope and the Five Keys to Shine Hope™ framework to help you create, maintain, and grow hope in the workplace. We give an overview of the framework, so you can then apply it to your career to activate hope at work. The course is available for individuals or to license to entire companies, to ensure all know the what, why, and how of hope.

You can learn more about the Hopeful Mindsets courses at www.hopecourses.com.

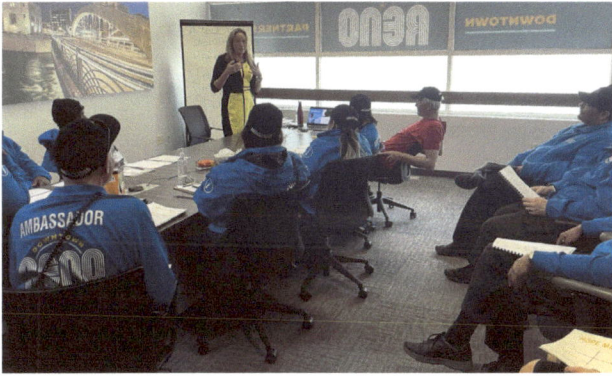

☼Hopeful Cities®

Hopeful Cities® is equipping cities around the world with the tools they need to create, maintain, and grow hope, citywide. Learn how you can activate hope in your community at www.hopefulcities.org.

☼ Hopeful Minds

Hopeful Minds® is programming for youth based on research that suggests hope is teachable (a skill). The aim is to equip students, teachers, and parents with the tools they need to define, learn, and grow Hopeful Minds in young kids. Learn more at www.hopefulminds.org.

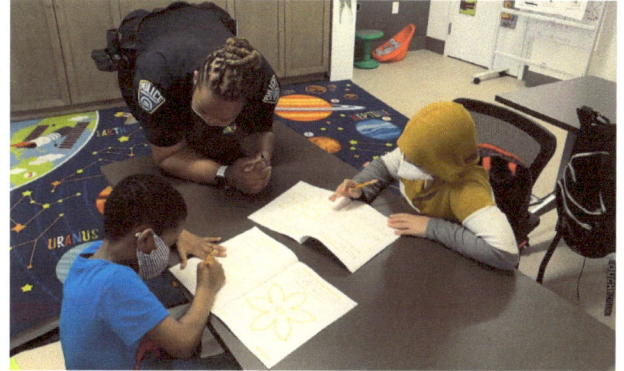

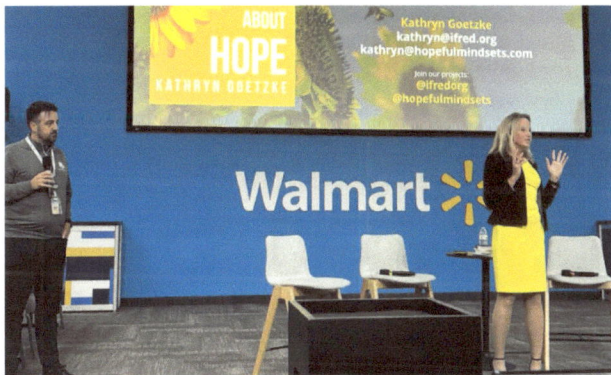

the shine hope™ company

The Shine Hope Company™ - Our mission is to improve lives globally by teaching scientifically informed and evidence-based methods to measure and cultivate hope. Learn how to activate hope in your life and community at www.theshinehopecompany.com.

If you are in need of support, you can find additional resources by visiting www.ifred.org/individual-support or scanning the QR Code.

HOPEFUL MINDSETS RESOURCES EXPERTS' BOOKS

Kathryn Goetzke, MBA
- The Biggest Little Book About Hope Second Edition

Dr. James Doty, MD
- Into the Magic Shop: A Neurosurgeon's Quest to Discover the Mysteries of the Brain and the Secrets of the Heart
- Mind Magic: The Neuroscience of Manifestation and How It Changes Everything

Dr. Chan Hellman, PhD
- Hope Rising: How the Science of Hope Can Change Your Life

Dr. Dan Tomasulo, PhD, TEP, MFA, MAPP
- Learned Hopefulness, The Power of Positivity to Overcome Depression
- The Positivity Effect: Simple CBT Skills to Transform Anxiety and Negativity into Optimism and Hope

Dr. Diane Dreher, PhD
- The Tao of Inner Peace

Ritu Riyat, MPH, MCHES
- The Stress Detox: Reduce Stress and Burnout in the Workplace

Dr. David B. Feldman, Ph.D
- Supersurvivors: The Surprising Link Between Suffering and Success

Dr. Steven C. Hayes, Ph.D. (Books in the last five years)
- Prosocial: Using evolutionary science to build productive, equitable, and collaborative groups.

Douglas Abrams
- Book of Joy
- Book of Hope

Dr. Robert Waldinger
- The Good Life: Lessons from the World's Longest Scientific Study of Happiness

Scan for complete list of expert's books.

This Coursebook was created by The Shine Hope Company. It is intended to accompany the Hopeful Mindsets on the College Campus Course, which can be purchased at www.hopecourses.com. The Hopeful Mindsets on the College Campus Course is not included in the purchase of this Coursebook.